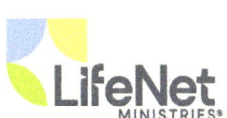

Life Launch

Youth Rite of Passage

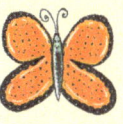

Diane Roblin-(Lee) Rutledge

Cheryl Rutledge

Rachelle Fletcher

LifeLaunch Softcover   978-1-896213-32-3
LifeLaunch E-book   978-1-896213-31-6
Date of Publishing - Oct. 1, 2023
Publisher - ByDesign Media *www.bydesignmedia.ca*
Copyright 2023 LifeNet Ministries Inc.
Author - Diane Roblin-Lee (Rutledge)
Research and development - Cheryl Rutledge
Contributing editor and distribution - Rachelle Fletcher
Cover and Inter design - Diane Roblin-Lee (Rutledge)

Disclaimer: The opinions expressed in this booklet are those of the authors and do not constitute part of the curriculum of any program beyond LifeLaunch. The development, preparation and publication of this work has been undertaken with great care. However, the authors, publisher, editors, and LifeNet Ministries Inc. associates are not responsible for any errors contained herein or for consequences that may ensue from use of materials or information contained in this work. The information contained herein is intended to assist individuals in personal growth and is distributed with the understanding that it does not constitute legal or medical advice. References to quoted sources are only as current as the date of the publication. Where any sourced material may have been inadequately referenced, the authors extend an apology. While every effort at adequate referencing has been taken, it is understood that research takes place over a lifetime, making it impossible to reference the source of every idea presented.

All rights reserved. No part of this publication may be reproduced, stored in a retrieval system, or transmitted in any form or by any means without prior permission of the copyright owner, LifeNet Ministries Inc.

byDesign
MEDIA

www.bydesignmedia.ca

Contents

Introduction — p. 5
1. Identity & Destiny Today — p. 7
2. Hanna ~ Self-Discovery Through Blessing — p. 13
3. Coming of Age Around the World — p. 17
4. The Importance of Rites of Passage — p. 23
5. The Power of Blessing — p. 27
6. The LifeLaunch Initiative — p. 31
7. Preparation — p. 33
8. Planning your LifeLaunch Celebration — p. 35
9. The Ceremony — p. 41
10. More Blessing — p. 43
11. For Further Reading — p. 45
12. Invitation Template — p. 47
13. Invitation List — p. 49–79
14. Guest Book — p. 81–109

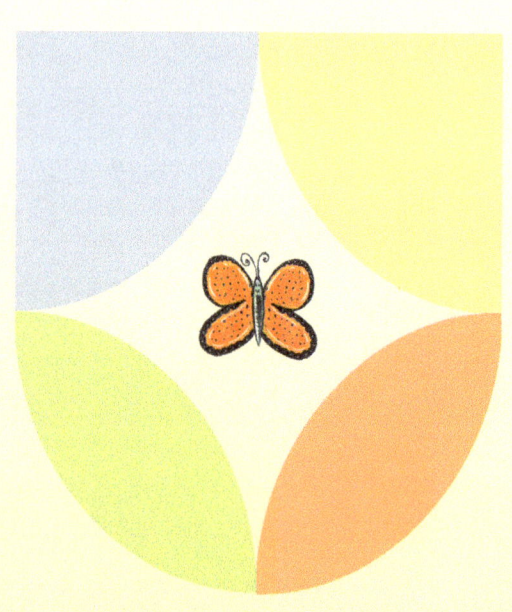

www.lifenet-lifelaunch.com

Introduction

LifeLaunch, the 21st century youth Rite of passage designed to transition young people successfully from childhood to adulthood, is an initiative of LifeNet Ministries Inc. The mandate of LifeNet is to restore hope to a generation so torn by the chaos of cultural revolution, that suicide reigns as the second leading cause of death for our oncoming generations, Gen Z and Gen Alpha.

But how did we get here? Why do our kids see death as the most expedient solution to their challenges? Do they really want to end their lives – or are they just desperate to find a way out of their pain? What holds them in this death-grip of struggle? How can we truly help them?

After participating at the funeral of a 12-year-old boy who had ended his life in Edmonton, Canada, Glen Rutledge[1] knew he had to allow God to change the trajectory of his life to reach similarly struggling children and teens. First developing TV programs *Circle Square* for children and *Inside Track* for teens, he went on to develop Circle Square Ranches across Canada (serving over 250,000 youth) and Teen Ranches in Australia. These served as a training ground and inspiration for more ranches in New Zealand, Scotland, Africa and elsewhere.

Glen was then given a vision for reaching out through the global internet with an initiative that came to be known as "LifeNet Ministries, Inc." Through LifeNet, that number of young people can potentially be reached in a day. A website, *www.lifenetministries.com* was built and an interactive, international call center was established to respond to callers.

---

1. Glen Rutledge was the co-founder (with David Mainse) of Crossroads Christian Communications Inc. and 100 Huntley Street.

The Troubling Question

In building LifeNet, the troubling question was, "How does one offer genuine, tangible hope to a generation faced with a future so different from traditional life-journeys?"

People used to offer hope in the same way they once received it:
"Just get a good education and you'll get a good job."
"Work hard and you'll have a nice home."
"Obey the law and you'll live a blameless life."
"Be nice and people will be nice to you."

And on it went…but it's not all necessarily true anymore. For Gen Z and Gen Alpha, everything appears to have changed: the economy, career expectations, gender issues, music, the focus of school curriculums, entertainment, methods of communication, opportunities, the definitions of marriage and family, the meaning of "friends" – and, most importantly, the position of today's world in relation to God's timeline.

While the one true and stable anchor is the Word of God, the traditional church has become so de-stabilized in today's society that finding ways to point kids to the simple message of God's love is challenging. With only two out of the under-thirty population reporting they believe church is important and 35 percent of Millennials reporting a strong aversion to it,[2] how do we (as the church) reach hearts with the eternal message without resorting to secular methods and compromising the amazing power of God's love? How do we offer hope that will resonate as true and foundational in the heart of a floundering adolescent today?

We are in a crisis. Finding workable answers to this question is a matter of life and death for thousands of families. The time is NOW to intervene on behalf of all subsequent generations or we could lose our opportunity. A LifeLaunch Rite of passage celebration won't fix everything, but it will help set the stage for a child to move forward with a strong sense of identity and destiny.

---

2. Eaton, S. "12 Reasons Millennials Are Over Church" Recklessly Alive. Sept. 29, 2016. *https://www.recklesslyalive.com/post/12-reasons-millennials-are-over-church* Accessed Sept. 3, 2023.

Chapter One

Identity & Destiny Today

The first step in discovering ways to reach out with authentic hope amid 21st century chaos, involves understanding the development of personal identity and a sense of destiny and how the process has changed for this generation.

Understanding what has changed opens doors for finding meaningful ways to transition our children through today's land mines of adolescence...to positive adulthood.

But some things haven't changed and so we must balance today with yesterday. Despite the glamorization of youth and today's unique challenges, adolescence has never been an easy season of life. It has always involved the hard work of establishing identity.

The questions, "Who am I?" Where do I fit in the world?" and "What do people think of me?" remain the drivers of adolescence despite the century.

What Has Changed?

Today's generation gap is the widest the world has ever seen. [3]

Historically, most children (according to God's design for humanity) had parents, an extended family and a caring community to help

---

3. Anderson, A., *Unscrambling the Millennial Paradox*, Crane MO, Defender Publishing, 2019, p. 18.

answer those questions and build paths of destiny and walls of protection around their lives.

Prior to the Industrial Revolution of the 1840's, almost every home consisted of a mother and a father who understood their responsibility to guide their children into successful adulthood. Home was expected to be the secure refuge where germination for personhood could flourish into healthy maturity.

But then came the post-WWII era of latch-key kids where Johnny and Suzy went to school with keys around their necks so they wouldn't lose them and find themselves unable to unlock the door when they got home. Gone were the days of bursting through the door after school, yelling, "Mom, I'm home!" Mom and Dad were both at work. The years of necessity (in some cases) gave way to other reasons for both parents working and the question, "Who am I," became, "Does anyone care who I am?"

Silence.

The Industrial Revolution gave way to the marvels of technology where the family sat with all chairs facing a box with moving pictures. Conversation became something observed as dialogue between actors. The question, "What do people think of me," became, "How do I measure up to the actors in the box?"

Silence.

Everyone became so absorbed with asking themselves the same question that they didn't notice the child's need for affirmation as he or she floundered. There was no button on the remote designated "parenting."

And then a new utensil was added in the dining-room. Where the family had once gathered over meals to chew over the happenings of the day, cell phones replaced the box and family TV viewing morphed into individual attention focused on personal devices. For many, the dining-room moved to the bedroom or any place one could sit and eat while focused on the cell phone, unencumbered by human interruption.

Silence.

Never before, in the history of the world have adolescents been so connected, yet so isolated – and the questions that drive them to establish or discover their identities remain.

When these questions, "Who am I?" "Where do I fit in the world?" and "What do people think of me?" are not answered in a constructive way in the developmental years, snippets of clues from offhand remarks, unwise judgments, manipulative input and sometimes cruel social media posts may serve as the only indicators a child absorbs about the nature of his or her identity.

When a parent fails to guard and guide the input imposed upon a child, or when a child finds him or herself vulnerable for whatever reason, and negative input finds its way into his or her psyche, walls of defense replace the walls of loving protection that should have guarded his or her heart. The child becomes wounded and wary of trusting anything posing as love.

Where bullying was once a relative rarity, unkindness and meanness have become increasingly normalized. Words of bullying, insensitivity or cruelty set up roadblocks, preventing the child from entering fully into his or her potential destiny. Fear of further damage to his or her identity locks up his or her heart and short-circuits his or her ability to interact in a loving way.

Vulnerability becomes scary. The possibility of experiencing further words of rejection, ridicule or resentment presents too great a risk to take.

Entertainment, new methods of communication, rejection of Christian foundations and changes in the focus of education are gradually changing the fabric of humanity.

The advent of Covid 19, with its isolationist mandates, separated adolescents from normal social interactions and participation in sports and groups that traditionally helped sort out strengths and weaknesses.

Rather that getting back to "normal" after the mandates were lifted, the accompanying cultural revolution, with a plethora of social media challenges, special interests lobbies, changes in social definitions and even changes in centuries-old usage of things like pronouns, dealt the death blow to "normalcy."

When the most basic markers of identity, like gender, began to be aggressively questioned, the anchors of humanity began to break loose and those not yet secure in who they were, found themselves adrift. It's no wonder nooses are being tied out of bedsheets and hoodies.

Our kids are staggering under the load society has imposed upon them and we must "do something!"

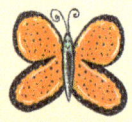

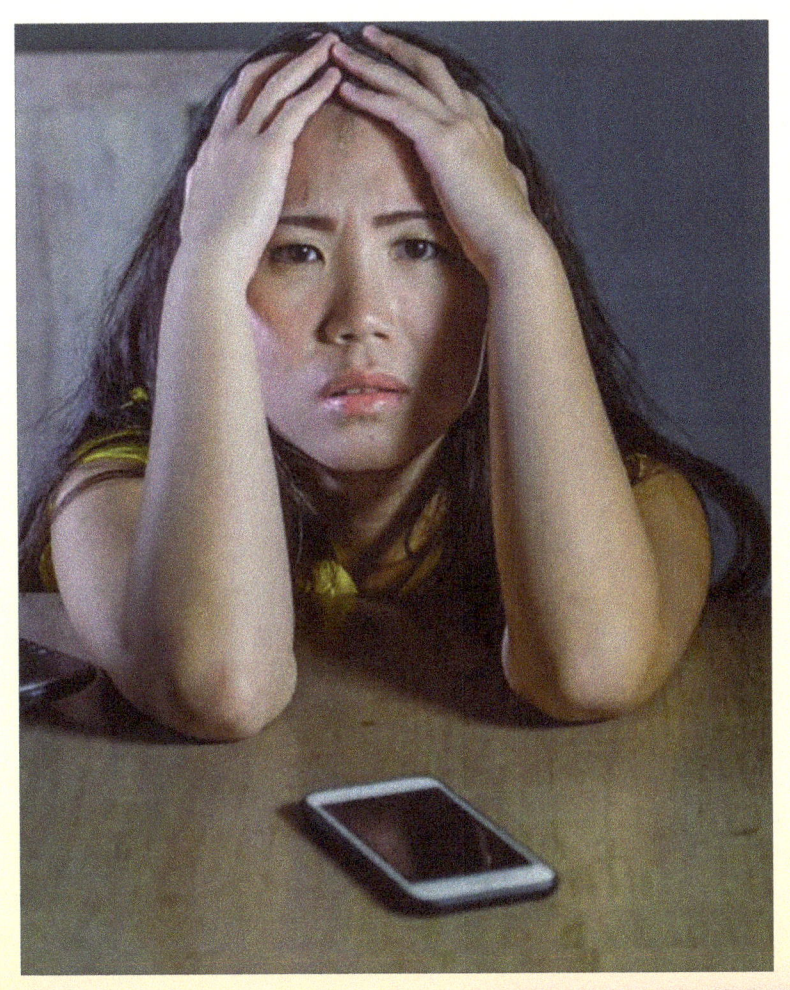

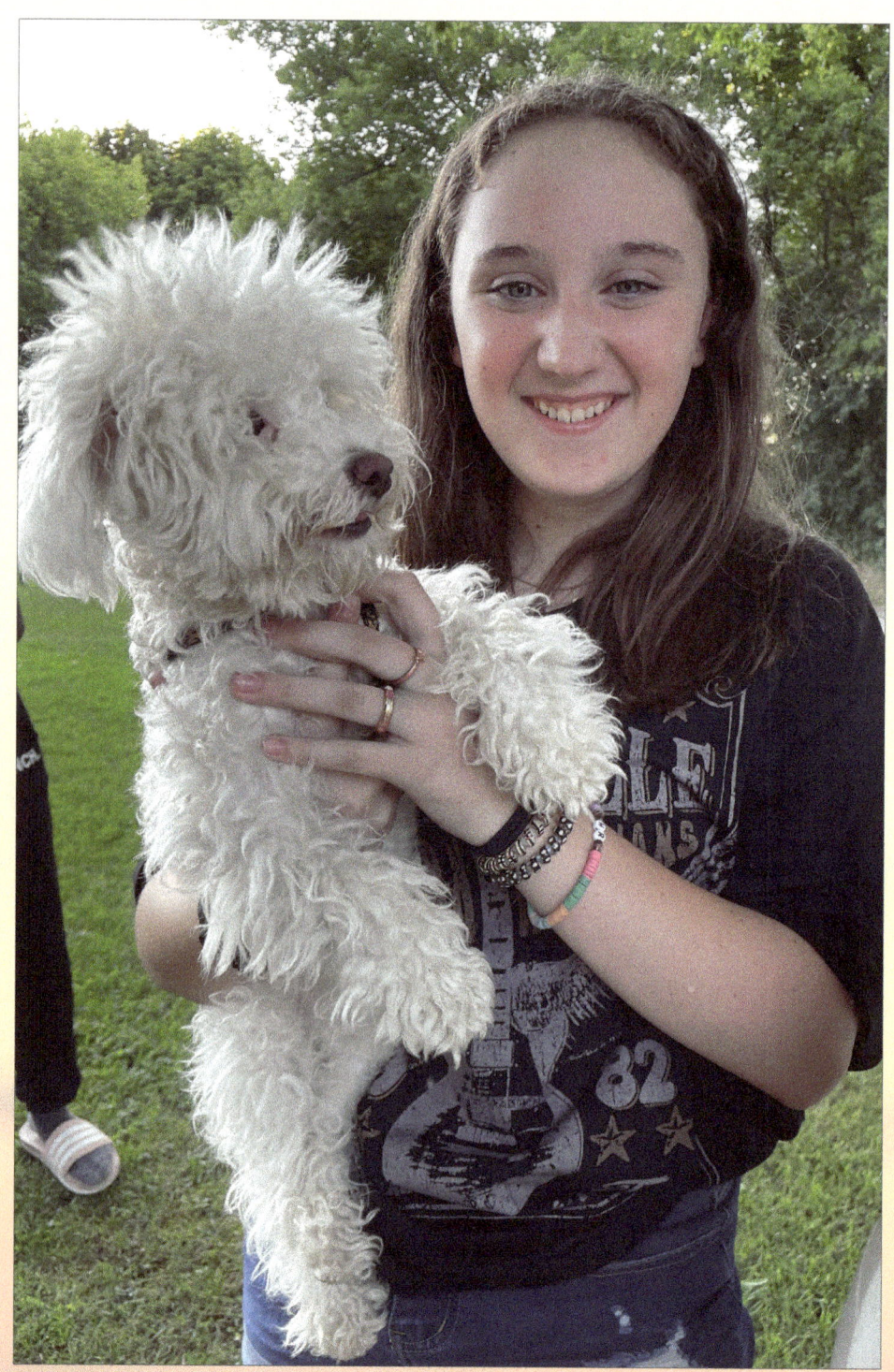

Hanna

Chapter Two

Hanna
Self-Discovery Through Blessing

Hanna's parents "did something."

If there is any such thing as a 'typical teenager,' Hanna would fill the bill. Faced with the same challenges as many other Gen Zs and Gen Alphas today, she struggled to find answers to the same questions that have always driven adolescents crossing the threshold from childhood to adulthood. "Who was she?" Where did she fit in the world?" and "What did people think of her?"

When she was about to turn 13, Hanna's family began to plan a special celebration for her. While they knew they couldn't wrap her in cotton batting and protect her from all the challenges that would come her way, they wanted to reassure her of all the wonderful potential they saw in her and give her as much confidence as possible for her journey ahead. While people may think their children understand their value, it's not always true. Hanna's parents knew she needed words and affirmations.

So they sent invitations to people who knew and loved her and asked eight of them to share their memories and hopes for her and speak words of blessing over her. They wanted their daughter to understand her significance in the lives of those around her.

When the special night arrived and the happy chatter of reunions subsided, Hanna was seated at a table in front of the podium. Yes, there were balloons, gifts and lots of chocolaty indulgences, but friends and family were gathered for a greater purpose than laughter and fun. They were there to participate in Hanna's Rite of passage.

Welcoming comments were followed by special music and guest after guest as they took their turns at the microphone. Each gave gifts of words that penetrated Hanna's heart as answers to her private questions concerning her emerging identity.

For anyone stealing glances Hanna's way, it was clear that something deep was happening. Although the audience couldn't see the tears, they saw her efforts to wipe them away at some point in almost every message. No one was concerned. They knew they were good tears – tears that were washing away any doubts of who she was and establishing her potential destiny and the value of her presence in this world.

But "blessing ceremonies" are not the norm in our world today. Our culture is devoid of meaningful Rites of Passage.

When I (Diane) was a child, there was no blessing ceremony, but a teacher's report contained the following assessment: "Diane is a most cooperative, capable, charming pupil." I tucked that in my heart as a definition of who I was. Later, when I was fooling around in high school, the vice principal, Mr. Roman, looked me straight in the eye and declared, "You'll never amount to anything."

Mr. Roman's words were powerful enough to have stayed in my mind for sixty years; but not powerful

Diane's Grade Three Report Card

enough to erase the words of Mrs. Crawford's blessing from my childhood. I had been defined as cooperative – and so I knew I needed to be cooperative. It was part of who I was, apparently. In like manner, I needed to be capable and charming – because that's who I was – not just because Mrs. Crawford said so, but because she planted the seed of potential she saw within me. Through activating the blessing, I was able to overcome the curse and 'amount to something.'

If there are no words of blessing over a child's life, overcoming words of cursing is much more difficult.

We need to fill our children up with blessing – not in flowery meaningless phrases – but by reassuring them of all the good potential we see and reminding them of God's promises over their lives. Positive affirmations are seeds of the marvelous destiny God has purposed for each individual.

While my blessing did not come by way of a formal ceremony, it was, none the less, a Rite of passage because it served to establish my identity within my heart. Interestingly, I saved that report and have kept it. It has accompanied me through all the moves and seasons of life.

Around the world, Rites of Passage have ushered the way for adolescents to transition into adulthood for centuries. Why have we in North America neglected such critical markers, the assurances that help young people to know who they are as they mature?

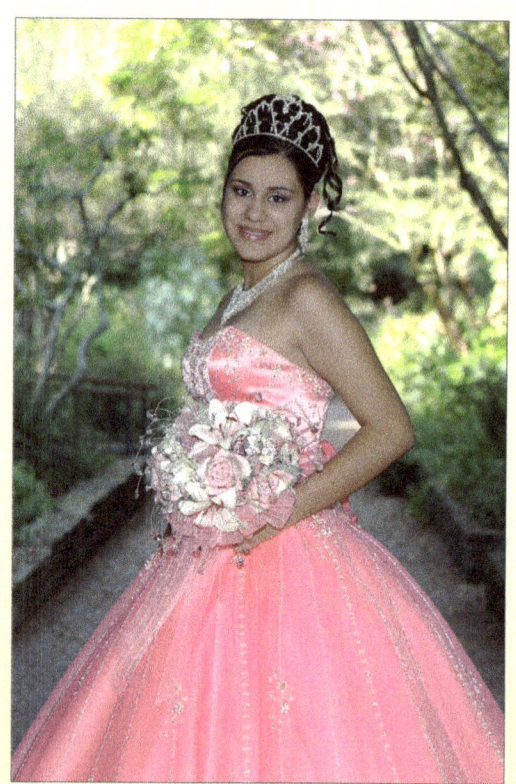

A 15-year-old Mexican girl celebrates her transition from childhood at her quinzianera fiesta.

Chapter Three

Coming of Age Around the World

North America is a continent of immigrants and indigenous peoples. Many of those who came here from other lands left behind a variety of cultural markers that established individual identities and enriched their history for generations.

Almost every culture on earth incorporates some form of a Rite of passage into adulthood except our own wewtern melting pot.

One clue regarding the absence of adolescent Rites of Passage in North America may be found in the British and French roots of most of the earliest settlers. For centuries, British children were to "be seen and not heard." Children were expected to follow established norms and not deviate from patterns of development. The thinking was that adulthood would happen despite variations in emotional needs – and surely everyone would understand his or her place in society without being told. Emotions were stifled through training to "keep a stiff upper lip." Heaven forbid that someone should display lack of intestinal fortitude by allowing an upper lip to tremble with emotion. Men grew up without tears or hugs, extending hands to shake rather than arms to embrace. Women packed their bags with social acceptability and emotional isolation and boarded the ships to emigrate to the new world.

Interestingly, many of the emigrants were not native to the British Isles, but were of Jewish origin, having fled Spain and the Iberian Peninsula to the British Isles during the Spanish Inquisition. Many of these carried with them the deeply entrenched traditions of blessing their families at Friday night Shabbat dinners and at the seven thresholds of life (conception, in utero, birth, infancy, puberty, marriage and old age) – but for the most part, these traditions did not spread from Jewish to Gentile communities. They were quietly observed behind ethnic doors.

Many of our indigenous people, those native to North America who found themselves integrated into modern society, discarded their old ways and the Rites of Passage that had served to transition children into adulthood. And so our society became sterile, immune to the understanding of the importance of stepping stones.

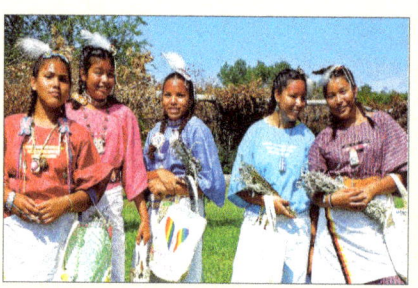

By the time immigrants began to arrive from countries all around the world, North America had become a cultural melting pot, where ethnic traditions and Rites of Passage that traditionally ushered children into adulthood, became indistinguishable elements of a faceless culture. With their focus on establishing new lives and blending into the new world, most immigrants dropped their treasured Rites of Passage.

While centuries old Rites of Passage became lost in North America, they remain rich in meaning in many foreign lands.

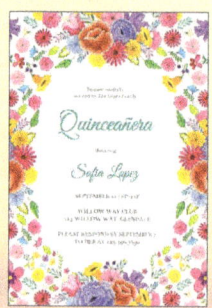

Latin countries celebrate Quinziana fiestas for young girls when they turn 15. Some of these celebrations are so elaborate that families go into debt providing wedding-dress quality finery, detailed programs and sumptuous multi-course dinners. They usually include a renewal of baptismal vows or recommittment to the girl's faith. Much planning and long anticipation is involved.

Vanatu is a country in the South Pacific Ocean. Comprised of around 80 separate islands and with a current population of under 350,000 people, it is one of the few remaining strongholds where indigenous culture and religion have remained mostly untouched by the effects of globalization. Their Rite of passage, signifying the transition from childhood to manhood, involves the practice of "land diving." Young boys start practicing at the age of eight, jumping head-first off a 20-foot-tall tower with only vines tied to his ankles. When they graduate to 100-foot-tall towers, the Rite of passage is complete and the jumper can enjoy recognition of his successfully achieved manhood.[4]

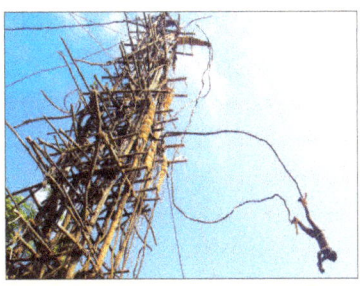

Growing up in Bali has its own unique challenges. Every Balinese youth, without exception, has to undergo the "tooth filling ceremony" as a Rite of passage into adulthood. The purpose of the ceremony is to affirm the belief that both good and evil exist in every person and symbolize rejection of the six negative inherent traits they recognize as the "Sad Ripu:" lust, greed, wrath, pride, jealousy, and intoxication (similar to the seven deadly sins of Christianity). "Ripu" means "enemy," as in "enemy of goodness." The ceremony involves symbolically filling the canines and incisors by lightly grazing the teeth with a piece of bamboo. The focus falls under the Balinese philosophy of harmonious relationships and is considered part of the responsibility of a parent to their child. As a culturally expected parental responsibility, there are no exceptions and, while there are no specific age requirements, the ceremony must be carried out prior to the wedding because it is this ceremony which transitions every Balinese youth into adulthood.[5]

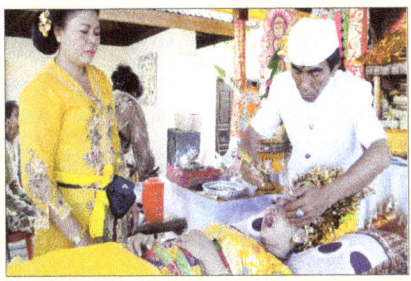

In Ethiopia, the Hamar tribe, mostly Muslim shepherds, live in camps consisting of several families. This tribe is known for its famous bull-jumping ceremony, the culmination of a three-day-long rite-of-

---

4. "Meet the Vanuatuan Land Divers: The Original Bungee Jumpers" April 14, 2022 by Joseph Sherwood *https://www.alittlebithuman.com/meet-the-vanuatuan-land-divers/* Accessed Aug. 1, 2023

5. "Tooth Filling, a Rite of passage" by a Balinese volunteer
https://volunteerprogramsbali.org/tooth-filing-a-Rite of passage/ Accessed Aug. 1, 2023

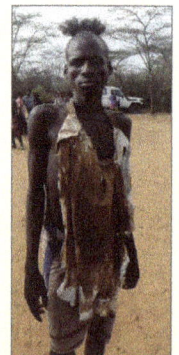 passage putting a young boy's valor and bravery to the test as he transitions into manhood. In order for him to be recognized and accepted as a man, he must be able to conquer his fears by running across the backs of seven to ten castrated bulls four times without falling. If successful, he is then sent to the elders and young men who bless him, shave his head and crown him with the title "Maza." It is a proud moment when the young boy proves his manhood. This ceremony is important because passing it qualifies him to own cattle, get married, and raise children. [6]

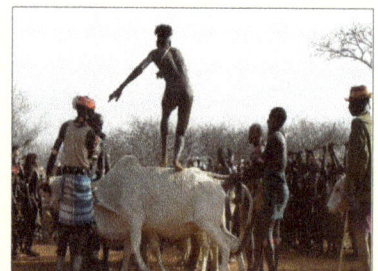

While land diving, tooth filling ceremonies and bull jumping may be foreign to this continent, the bar and bat mitzvahs of Jewish communities are more familiar, and therefore more acceptable, to western society with its Judeo-Christian roots.

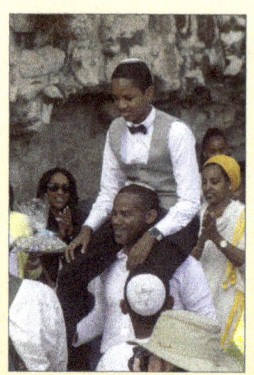 A Jewish boy becomes a man in terms of religious responsibility at the age of 13. Although bar mitzvah ceremonies weren't in practice until the middle ages, the Rite of passage was recognized in ancient times. Bat mitzvahs, celebrated for girls at the age of 12, emerged as the feminine equivalent to the male status in the 20th century. Today's versions generally involve ceremonies but the term implies a status of religious responsibility rather than a ceremony.

The story of the young Jewish Jesus amazing priests in the temple, referenced their recognition of him as a knowledgeable, religiously responsible student of the Torah (God's instructions on how to live). While the bar mitvah ceremony was not an ancient rite, this example of Jesus as a

---

6. "The Culture Behind the Bull Jumping Ceremony," Absolute Ethiopia Tours *https://absoluteethiopia.com/the-culture-behind-the-bull-jumping-ceremony/* Accessed August 1, 2023

young boy in the Temple confirmed the God-ordained Rite of passage for adolescents. Young boys of the day would go with their fathers to interview priests considering their rules and expectations, called "yokes." [7]The challenge was to find one suitable as a mentor for each particular boy. When the student completed the requirements of the priest, he (or she) received recognition of religious status (bar/bat mitzvah).

Because they have retained this God-ordained Rite of passage for adolescents, and continue to bless their sons and daughters at Friday night Shabbat (Sabbath) dinners and at other stages of their development, Jewish parents have had tools for ushering their children over thresholds of life. Jewish adolescents are recognized as having a strong sense of their identity as they journey through their teens.

In general, however, North American adolescents have been left without the ceremonies and customs through which they traditionally received impartations and affirmations of their identity at special junctures of their lives.

It's not that North American parents have failed their children; it's just that, in large part, they have forgotten the tools God gave them to usher their offspring through the chaos of this life.

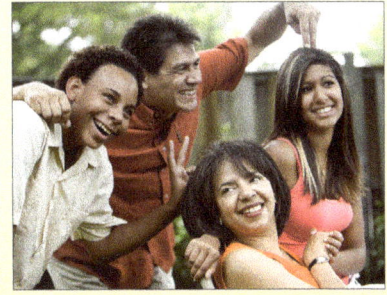

It's obvious from the variety of Rites of Passage embedded in almost every culture that there is an innate understanding of the importance of recognizing and assisting young people over thresholds. God made each child different and understanding who we are as individuals is critical. Every child has unique giftings, talents and destiny. When these are recognized by the community that surrounds a child, it makes it easier for the child to move forward with confidence in his or her identity towards his or her destiny.

---

7. When encouraging us to choose Him as our High Priest as we transition from spiritual immaturity to spiritual maturity, Jesus said, *"Come to Me all you who labor and are heavy laden, and I will give you rest. Take My yoke upon you, and learn from Me, for I am gentle and lowly in heart, and you will find rest for your soul. For My yoke is easy and My burden is light"* (Matthew 28:30).

The dark forces of today have tried to destroy the identities of our children through crazy rhetoric and insane narratives, but the stifling of identity has *always* been a tool of destructive forces.

A good example of this dark struggle can be found in the Book of Daniel in the story of Shadrach, Meshach, and Abednego, the young men who survived Nebuchadnezzar's fiery furnace. Many people don't know that those were not their real names. King Nebuchadnezzar (who was determined that they should serve pagan gods instead of their Most High God) changed their names. He wanted to take away their identity and make them slaves to paganism. Hananiah (meaning "God is gracious") became Shadrach (meaning "command of the moon god). Mishael (meaning "who is God") became Meshach (meaning "who is Aku"). Azariah (meaning "God has helped") became Abednego (which means "slave of the god Nebo).[8]

These boys had been anointed by God for His purposes, but when they refused to bow to evil, the enemy tried to take them out by changing their names and throwing them into the worst possible situation. Nevertheless, they had the mark of the Holy Spirit on them, so it didn't work. Satan will always try to throw our children into the worst circumstances and rob them of understanding who they really are, but if they know their identity and who they are as children of the Most High God, it won't work. Efforts to discourage them will disappear through victory. The true identities of Hananiah, Mishael and Azariah were established through centuries because they were proven by God's supernatural, saving power.

God forbid that any of our children should have to discover or prove their identities through surviving fire, but it's the same God who protected those three young men who wants to protect our children today through their journey into adulthood.

But why do they need a ceremony?

---

8. Reynolds, D., "What is the Meaning of the Names Shadrach,Meshach, and Abednego," https://www.enotes.com/homework-help/what-is-the-meaning-of-the-names-shadrach-meshach-2375930, Accessed August 20, 2023.

Chapter Four

The Importance of Rites of Passage

"A Rite of passage is a ceremony or ritual of the passage which occurs when an individual leaves one group to enter another. It involves a significant change of status in society."[9]

Birth, transitioning to adulthood, marriage, divorce parenthood, old age and death all involve crossing thresholds from one human condition to another. Some involve ceremonies, while others pass unmarked except for community recognition of status.

D. A. Lertzman, in his work, *Rediscovering Rites of Passage,* says: "When these times of transition are marked, ritualized, witnessed, and supported, it creates a kind of experiential map of self-development. Without proper Rites of Passage, people can become disoriented and lose their way on life's journey."[10]

What happens when Rites of Passage are ignored and rituals fall by the wayside? Whether ignored or acknowledged, the life-events still happen and may morph into attempts at self-initiation. According to psychologists, this may involve the testing of one's extreme limits of feelings and behaviors (without assistance or accountability) by way of substance abuse or dangerous activities.[11]

---

9. Rite of passage. (2023, July 2). In Wikipedia. https://en.wikipedia.org/wiki/Rite_of_passage, Accessed August 3, 2023

10. Lertzman, D. A. 2002. Rediscovering Rites of Passage: education, transformation, and the transition to sustainability. Conservation Ecology 5(2): 30. [online] URL: http://www.consecol.org/vol5/iss2/art30/

11. Ibid.

When Rites of Passage are rediscovered and observed in whatever way, dangerous self-initiations may be avoided and memories can be made that serve both the initiate and the family/community in an inspirational way, cementing an "increased sense of purpose and place in the world for the young person."[12]

A Rite of passage to adulthood always includes three stages:
1) Moving away from childhood and the system that supported one's childhood.
2) Crossing the threshold where one is neither child nor adult. This stage varies in duration, according to the individual and circumstances. It is made more definitive with a planned Rite of passage.
3) Emerging into the responsibilities and recognition of adulthood. This is the point at which the child steps into expectations of progressive maturity with its rights, responsibilities and privileges. It requires some measurement of proving oneself, through whatever personal, cultural, familial or community requirements are available.

The Benefits of Rites of Passage for Mental Health

With so much emphasis on mental health in this generation, it's helpful to consider the benefits of youth Rites of Passage for mental health.

"Rites of Passage support young people in the process of becoming whole, productive and contributing members of the family and community.
"Young persons come out of the experience with a new and empowering story that helps them take responsibility for the decisions that set the course of their future.
"Young persons are supported while creating the story of who they are and the kind of life they want to build based on the exploration of their own personal values.
"Through this self-exploration, initiates emerge with a stronger

---

12. Ibidem.

sense of personal responsibility for all aspects of their lives, taking full responsibility for their own actions as an adult.

"If Rites of Passage help a young person to navigate safely from childhood into adulthood, find purpose/meaning in life, become more self-confident and become an active and responsible member of his/her community and society, they ultimately support positive mental health.

"Positive mental health, according to WHO, is a state of wellbeing in which the individual recognizes his or her own abilities, can manage the normal stresses of life, can work effectively, and is able to play a role in his or her community."[13]

The proven (over centuries) benefits of Rites of Passage make one wonder why a society as progressive, civilized and blessed as North America would not have incorporated them into our culture. Could it be because North American culture, itself, is an adolescent society still experiencing its own form of growing pains? If so, is it not to the detriment of those growing up within it? Is it not time to recognize a missing key element and reinstate it?

A Rite of passage may not be the defining instrument to wipe away all the challenges our young people face today, but solid solutions generally emerge as the sum of all good things.

Taking a fresh approach to the way we launch our children into adulthood, by establishing a new North American Rite of passage for them, is a good thing.

It's all about blessing our kids over the threshold!

Ceremonies bring closure to certain seasons of life and welcome new ones. Just as a wedding brings closure to the single life and opens the door for creating a new family unit, a rite of passage around the time of puberty closes the door on childhood and releases the young person into confident manhood or womanhood.

---

13. Falanga, Barbara Rodi, "Rites of Passage and Positive Mental Health of Young People" *https://positivementalhealth.eu/2020/12/22/Rites of Passage-and-positive-mental-health-of-young-people/* Accessed Aug. 4, 2023

There is very little gender confusion in cultures where the deep questions of identity are settled at the time of puberty through the loving impartation of blessing through a parent.[14] When gender is settled, there is no more need to prove manhood or womanhood to anyone. Understanding oneself brings peace to the soul.

Much of today's in-your-face sexual immorality is the fruit of constant striving to prove masculinity or femininity – or the flip side of either. A girl who has never been blessed by her parents will search elsewhere for blessing, thinking it will be found as response to her sexuality. Sexual conquest is the journey travelled by many young men in search of proof of their identity.[15]

Age of Transition

The feeling of being a child or an adult is not a matter of age; it's dependent on when a young person is ready for an emotional release into adulthood.[16] That's why God intended for everyone to experience a powerful release into adulthood through ceremonial blessing.[17]

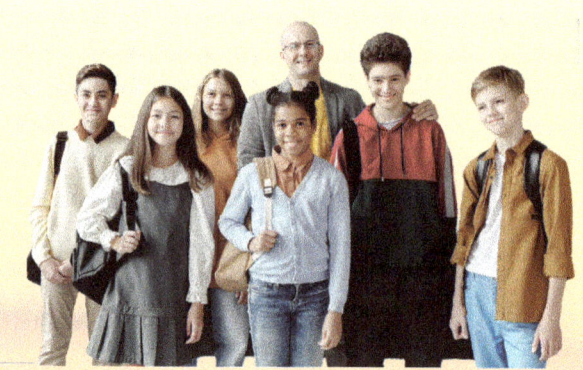

14. Hill, C., *Bar Barakah*, Family Foundations Publishing, Box 320, Littleton CO 80160, p. 8.

15. Ibid, p. 15.

16. Ibidem, p.14

17. Ibidem, p. 14

Chapter Five

The Power of Blessing

No one had to tell Esau and Jacob about the importance of the blessing of their father, Isaac. Most people are familiar with the story of the lengths to which their mother, Rebecca, went to make sure her youngest, favorite son Jacob received his father's blessing – when it would normally have gone to her eldest son, Esau. When Esau discovered the blessing had been stolen from him, "he cried with an exceedingly great and bitter cry."[18]

The blessing carried with it the empowerment to prosper, not only in terms of economic success, but in terms of doing well in all areas of life. When a father laid his hands on the head of his son and imparted his blessing, he imparted to him the ability to do well and succeed in his life purpose, to have a pleasant, fulfilling journey.

The original Hebrew word translated as "Bless" is the verb "Baruch," meaning "to empower to prosper."

Blessing isn't something that ended with antiquity. We hear of it today in the traditions of a variety of groups but the understanding of its power has been diminished through lack of understanding or through the enshrouding of dusty tradition.

Words have power. Proverbs 18:21 reads, *"Death and life are in the power of the tongue, and those who love it will eat its fruits."*

---

18. Genesis 27:34-36, 41)

God made a covenant with Abraham, the power of which extends to us today. "...*I will bless you and make your name great, so that you will be a blessing. I will bless those who bless you, and him who dishonors you I will curse...*" (Genesis 12:2-3)

"Blessing is God's primary mechanism of imparting His message of identity and destiny into (one's) life...A simple definition of blessing is, 'To receive, accept, ascribe high value to, and consider the person a success.'"[19]

Smalley and Trent, in their book, *The Blessing*,[20] define the blessing that should be imparted through parents or guardians as containing five key elements:
- Meaningful touch
- A spoken message
- The attachment of high value to the one being blessed
- The picturing of a special future for the one being blessed
- An active commitment to fulfill the blessing.

Both historically and today, the vehicle God designed to impart blessing was/is the family.

It is through the life, death, resurrection and example of Jesus Christ, that God is intent on blessing His creation - but we must give Him the opportunity and the recognition to do so.

The lines of division between good and evil are being drawn with more clarity than ever before in history. If we don't serve to strengthen our young people through blessing, agents of Satan will serve to destroy their identity and destiny. Without blessing, our children will be left to flounder through years of searching for clues to who they are, where they fit in the world and what people think of them. They may spend a lifetime trying to prove their value through getting enough money, looking good enough, achieving high goals or doing something great.

19. Hill, Craig, The Ancient Paths, Family Foundations International, Box 320, Littleton, Colorado 80160, 1992 ISBN 1-881189-01-5, p.27.

20. Smalley, Gary and Trent, John, "The Blessing," Thomas Neilsen, Nashville, USA, 1986, ISBN 9780849946370.

But it's never enough. Money can vanish in a day and wrinkles are inevitable. Blessing establishes transcendant value, value that supercedes circumstances. Blessing establishes and enables the blessed person to rest in the knowledge that he or she is valued.

Blessing vs Behavior

There are those who will hesitate to bless a child who is behaving badly; but identity and behavior are not fused issues. Confusion happens when a parent fears that if he or she blesses a child, the behavior will be condoned. Behavior needs to be disciplined but a primary root of teen rebellion is lack of parental blessing.[21]

We bless the person and discipline the behavior.

A prime example of separation of blessing and behavior is found in Romans 5:8: *"...but God shows his love for us in that while we were still sinners, Christ died for us."* God didn't wait for us to be perfect before He blessed us; He died for us.

Blessing vs Control

Are we saying parents can control the destiny of a child through blessing? It's not about control. Unfortunately, all some people have known is control and they mistake it for parenting.

If we take our cues from Scripture, it's obvious that God doesn't parent us via control. He gave us free will – the freedom to make our own life choices. But choices come with good or bad consequences. Consistency in follow-through with reasonable, logical consequences makes for parenting with peace in the home.

Governing a child with loving authority is called, "parenting." Rebellion is the fruit of control but respect is the fruit of blessing with loving authority.

---

21. Anderson, A., *Unscrambling the Millennial Paradox*, Crane MO, Defender Publishing, 2019, p. 23.

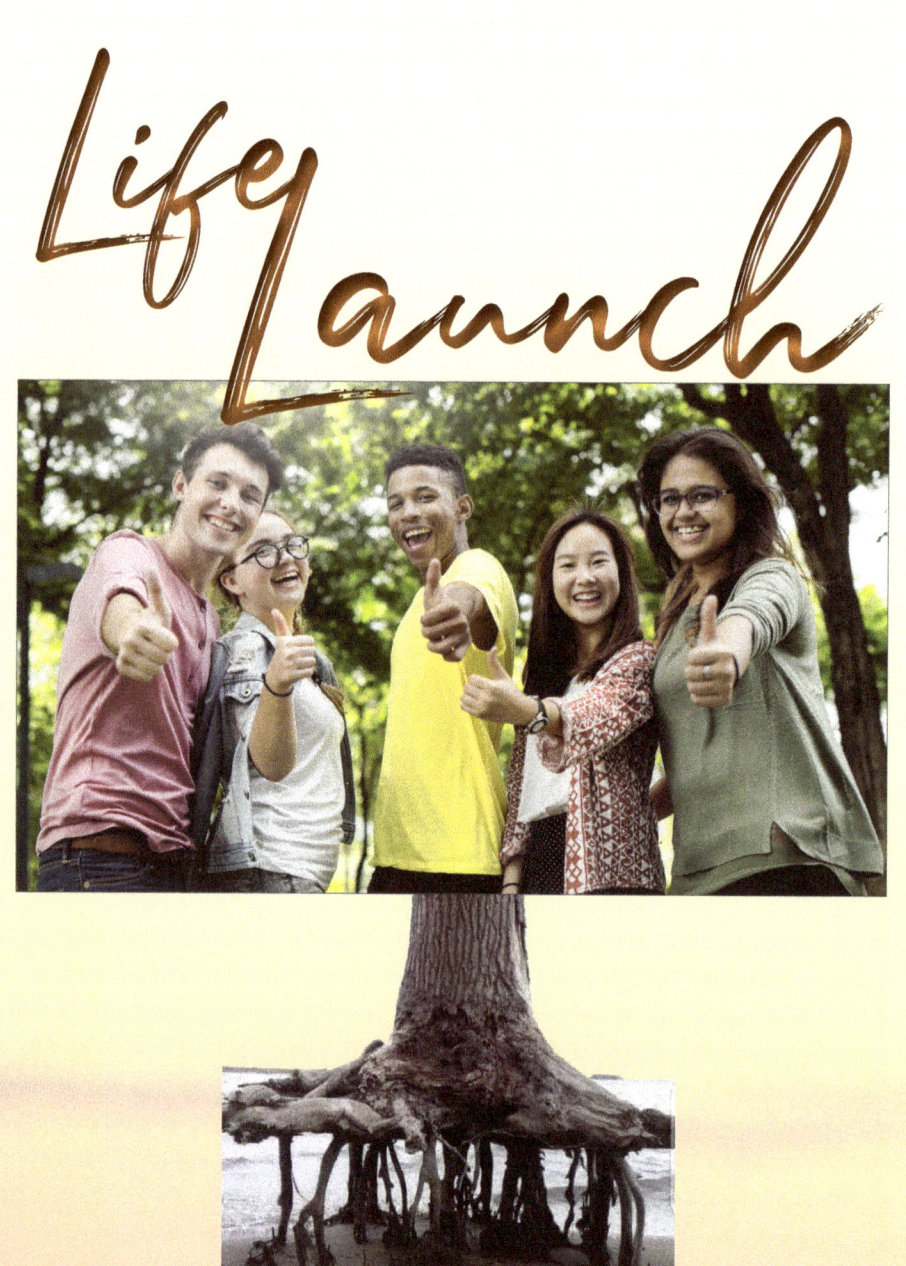

Life Launch

Rooted in the Promises and Purposes of God

Chapter Six

The LifeLaunch Initiative

The "LifeLaunch" initiative offers a template for ushering young people from childhood to a confident adulthood.

LifeLaunch fills the void as a North American Rite of passage to assure adolescents of their potential, destiny and value to the world. It is a call to re-affirm the order of God's plan for His Creation, to return to the things in life that worked. Jeremiah 6:16 speaks of finding rest for our souls when we walk in His ways.

> *Thus says the Lord:*
> *"Stand by the roads, and look,*
> *and ask for the ancient paths,*
> *where the good way is; and walk in it,*
> *and find rest for your souls.*
> *But they said, 'We will not walk in it.'*

We have experience the results of not walking in God's ways. Our children may not understand it, but they are crying out for us to return to His paths for their benefit.

With suicide raging as the second leading cause of death among our teens, we know we can't save every child, but we believe that by helping equip Christian families with tools to strengthen their adolescents, some teens will catch a hitherto elusive glimpse of hope and resist the urge to end their lives; others, who get excited about God's love, will share it with struggling friends and kids they know.

The goal is to establish the understanding of a young person's value through blessing.

LifeLaunch is a vehicle for preparing a young person to fulfill his or her destiny – not to just get a job. It is a tool for putting questions of significance and purpose to rest, to bypass the never-ending treadmill of the search for significance through revelation and confirmation of identity.

These issues will be settled through a powerful, genuine impartation of blessing through parents, guardians and community.

What About Single Parents?

The tragedy of death, divorce or separation has left many homes short of God's design for two-parent families. This is where the community can step up and offer blessing for a child.

At LifeNet, we believe that if every solid family would take responsibility for one child not their own, this world would be a different place.

Church or Community Initiatives

Where it's obvious that a child is not going to have the opportunity to be launched across the threshold from childhood to the beginning of adulthood by his or her family, it's a wonderful opportunity for the church or community to step up to the plate and bless the life of a young person in a very meaningful way. Whether planned individually or as a group event, it could make all the difference in a teen journey.

Paying it Forward

A blessed teen may want to reach out to friends who won't have the experience of blessing unless he or she takes the initiative and finds a way to make it happen. Blessing and affirmation don't always have to come through adult channels.

The LifeLaunch Rite of Passage plan is included on the "Family Connect" page of our LifeNet Ministries website www.lifenetministries.com or www.LifeNet4Hope.com

Chapter Seven

Preparation

We suggest that you start preparing your child for his or her Rite of passage anywhere from a year to six months prior to the special event, usually prior to the 12th or 13th birthday; but the best indicator of timing is the point at which a parent sees evidence of some emotional maturity, interest in issues of sex and thoughts of long-time goals. Around the time of puberty, most children are still open to receiving instruction and guidance and enjoy spending time with their family.

Discuss the importance of this threshold in terms of transitioning from childhood into the first stages of adulthood with the significance of its new responsibilities, freedoms and recognition of developing maturity.

Beyond discussions of what this will mean in day to day living, impart to your child a sense of God's plans and purposes for his or her life. Explore the giftings and talents that have become evident through childhood and focus on those as markers for the journey ahead. Whatever the call God has on his or her life, He will have planted tools within your young person to fulfill His wonderful, unique purposes for each one.

Teach your child about the power of blessing and the importance of the words spoken over his or her life. Prepare him or her to overcome negative words (that can manifest as curses) that will invariably be spoken here and there through life, with the words of blessing which will be spoken at the Rite of passage event and on throughout life.

Consider developing a family mission statement to guide and and anchor your family. Build your roots deep so that when storms come, you can face them together with strength.

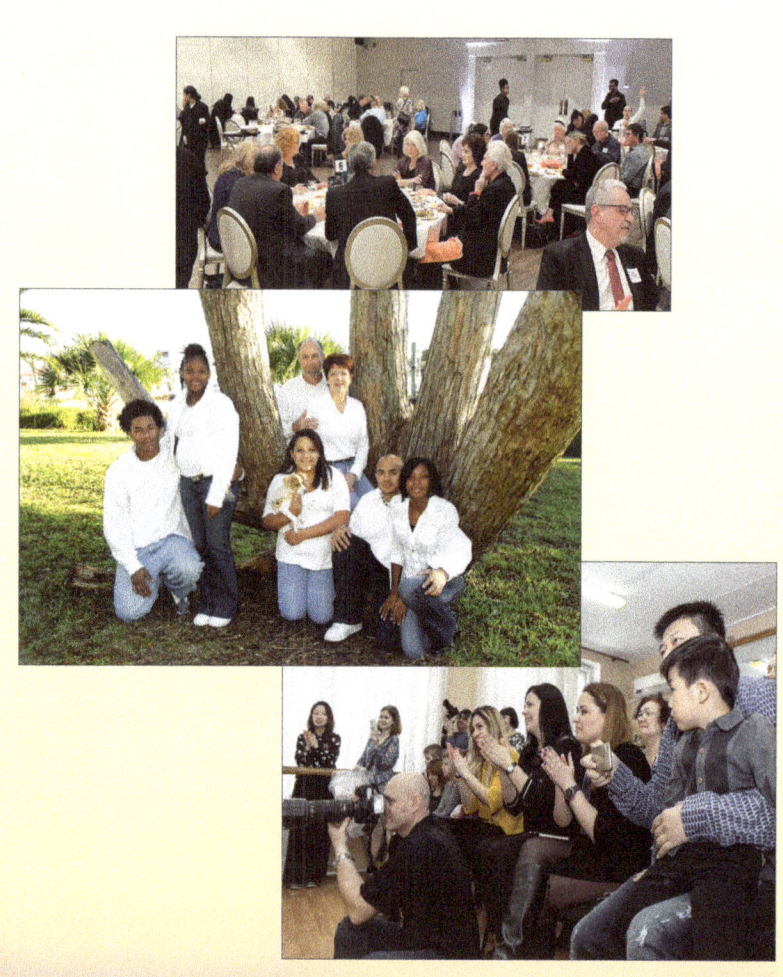

Chapter Eight

Planning

The LifeLaunch blessing celebration should be an honouring experience to God, your young person and to all those involved in the celebration as participants or guests.

The following is a suggested guide for planning your LifeLaunch rite of passage.

Involve God

If you involve the Holy Spirit in your plans, you'll be amazed at how they will flow. Everything will feel 'right.' He is the one who knows your young person most intimately and what elements to include that will touch his or her heart most deeply.

Involve Your Young Person

Be sure to involve your young person in the planning. Make it a fun time of choosing invitations. decorating, and making food, music and venue choices. Creating the guest and speaker list together will help ensure eager anticipation of the event.

Budget

Expense issues are entirely individual. A LifeLaunch celebration can range anywhere from a simple home celebration to an elaborate fiesta with all the trimmings. The point is to make it meaningful to the heart of your young person. It's not about impressing your neighbour; it's about helping your child to transition from childhood, over the threshold into successful teen and adult years. It's about the heart, not the material display. If your budget allows and you're able to splurge on things your young person would enjoy, that's wonderful – but don't allow budget restraints to prevent the planning of a gathering of friends and family to launch your young person.

Invitations

As you consider the invitation list (see the Invitation Workbook section), consider carefully the people who have mentored or nurtured your child in a variety of ways. These could include peers who have been a positive influence. As people respond to your invitation (See Invitation Template on p. 38), be sure to record their response under the "Coming" column. Invitations should typically be out a month or two prior to the event. RSVPs should be received two weeks prior to the event to help you finalize details. Encourage those who are unable to attend to write letters of blessing to your young person. They will be cherished.

Participants in the Ceremony

We suggest inviting eight to ten participants (including parents) to share memories, insights or special words concerning your child. This will be the main body of the ceremony. The purpose is to pour lasting affirmation of value into your child to provide sure footing for the way ahead. These people could be chosen from a variety of aspects of your child's life: perhaps relatives from both sides of the family (if available), a youth pastor, a teacher, a coach, a music of dance teacher, an employer, a close family friend or a leader from a club or activity in which your child is involved. Parents generally MC the ceremony, welcoming guests at the beginning and thanking them for coming at the close. The participants should be chosen for their obvious recognition of giftings, abilities or potential in your child.

As an example, in Hanna's case (Chapter Two), Hanna was very shy and unsure of herself until an aunt saw beyond her immaturity to her potential. When Hanna opted to participate behind the scenes in a church drama, her Aunt Deb (who was directing the play) encouraged her to take one of the lead roles (which Hanna did). As her aunt walked her through her fear to help her stretch and grow, Hanna nailed the part and went on to participate in other dramas to exercise her God-given acting abilities. Through that encouragement, she went on to try out for cheer leading in her community sports program and won a place on the cheer squad – a far cry from the shy child she once was. At Hanna's rite of passage, her aunt was one of the participants, reaffirming the growth and promise she had witnessed in Hanna, and encouraging her to develop the talents and giftings that had become evident through daring to step out and take part in the drama. She confirmed and affirmed the stirrings of confidence Hanna had experienced. She turned her taste of success into an appetite for experiencing more successes in life. Her words were a major element in giving Hanna the confidence to try out and make the cheer squad. They were foundational.

Each guest who is invited to share should be prompted in the purpose of his or her words. It's not just a party for sharing funny stories (although those will add a wonderful element of humour); it's an opportunity to speak words of declaration, purpose and value into your child's life. It's an opportunity for recognized giftings to be established through words of confirmation and affirmation.

Plan the Seating at the Venue

Planning for table and seating set-up can be as detailed or casual as you like. Some may incorporate a seating plan which will be clearly visible to arriving guests, while others may be happy to have guests seat themselves. Whether you organize the guests or not, there needs to be a clearly defined place for the young guest of honour at the front, either in a solitary chair facing the podium where participants will speak, or at a table surrounded by key figures in his or her life (generally immediate family).

Frame the Event with Scripture

Choose a Scripture to read in the ceremony that will be meaningful for your young person. Incorporating some of the promises of God lays the most solid foundation for your young person moving forward in life.

We suggest incorporating Jeremiah 29:11 at some point to assure your young person of the greater plans and purposes God has ahead for him or her. *"I know the plans I have for you, declares the Lord, plans for welfare and not for evil, to give you a future and a hope."*[1]

The 13th Chapter of Judges tells the story of Samson, whose father, Manoah asked, *"What is to be the child's manner of life, and what is his mission?"*[2]

Photo Overview of Childhood

Consider organizing an digitizing photos of your child's history and childhood for a montage screen presentation.

Video Recording

Consider appointing someone to video the entire event. This will be a very emotional, at times overwhelming, experience for your teen and it will be impossible to absorb all its details at the time. Videoing it will provide a rich opportunity to appreciate it in its fullness over the days and years ahead.

Make sure all the microphones, cords and other equipment are in working order prior to the event.

---

1. ESV
2. ESV

Live Streaming

For those unable to attend the event for reasons of distance, illness or prior committments, making it available via live streaming is a wonderful option. If you make this option available, make it known to those who will need it and make sure all your technical ducks are in a row.

Music

Music is more important to memory than many people understand. While poetry or scripture may be difficult to memorize on their own, when lyrics are arranged with melody, they are more easily fastened to memory. If you include special music, including powerful worship songs in your ceremony, every time your child hears those songs throughout his or her life, memories of the spoken blessings will wash over his or her mind. Even when they're not being physically played or sung, God can spark a replay in his or her mind, reaffirming the personal blessing.

The Guestbook

While not all guests will be asked to share publicly, the included LifeLaunch Guestbook provides an opportunity for everyone to share lasting words of encouragement, prophetic words, etc., that will serve as seeds for healthy development and growth.

A Token of Remembrance

Even if your budget is small, consider presenting your child with a token of remembrance of his or her LifeLaunch rite of passage – perhaps a bracelet, a pendant, an inscribed Bible, a memory book or whatever would bring symbolic remembrance of his or her rite of passage.

Gifts

Because many of the guests will want to bring gifts or cards, it's important to designate a table with a basket for cards, as the "Gift Table." Greeters should be able to direct those arriving with gifts to the table as they arrive.

p. 40

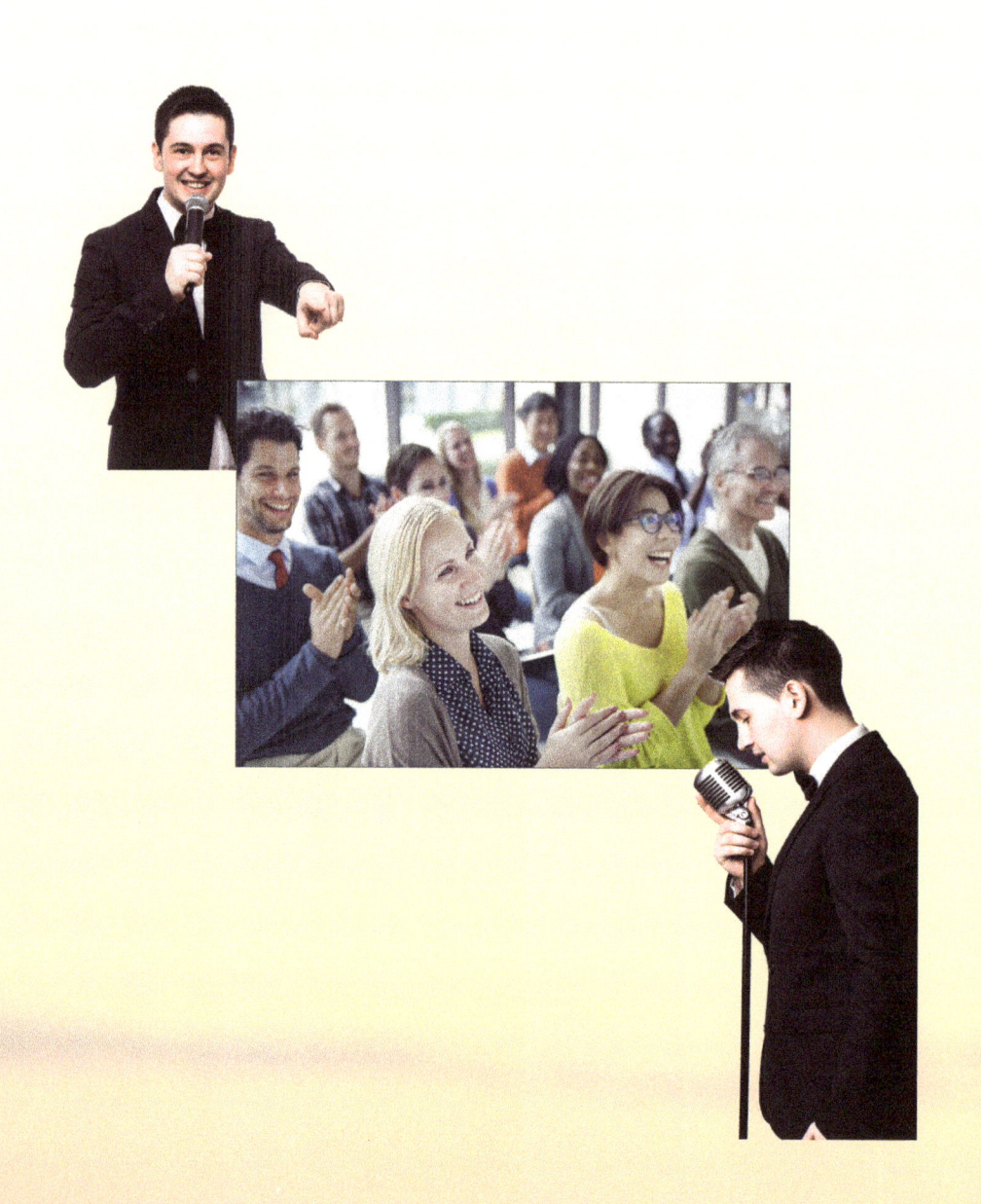

Chapter Nine

The Ceremony

The following are a few suggestions designed to be helpful in planning the LifeLaunch ceremony for your teen.

1. Welcome your guests as individually as possible as they arrive and as a group welcome to signal the start of your program. If you are live-streaming, extend the welcome to your online guests.

2. No matter what the degree of formality of your event, opening in prayer will set the tone and importance of the agenda to follow. If you're asking God to bless your young person, it helps to invite His presence. :)

3. Photo montage of history and childhood projected on screen.

4. Create an atmosphere of honour with worship music that will be meaningful to your teen. Depending on budget, resources and musical abilities your friends or family may have, your contemplative time of worship can be more or less elaborate. Whether through the aid of technology or a live band, this will be an important time of setting the stage for what is to follow.

5. Have someone read the chosen Scripture.

6. The parent or guardian (whoever is the master of ceremonies) will typically begin with a few words about the young person being celebrated.

7. Words of blessing from designated participants.

8. Perhaps more special music.

9. Seal up this time of blessing with prayer to establish what has been spoken.

Having the Aaronic Blessing spoken over your teen at this time (perhaps by a grandparent or parent) is a powerful finalization of the ceremony. These were the words of God and they carry the ultimate in authority and blessing.

The Lord bless you and keep you.
The Lord make his face to shine upon you and be gracious to you.
The Lord lift up his countenance upon you and give you peace.
(Numbers 6:24-26)[3]

10. Master of ceremonies thanks the participants and invites guests to enjoy a time together over dinner or goodies.

11. Reception

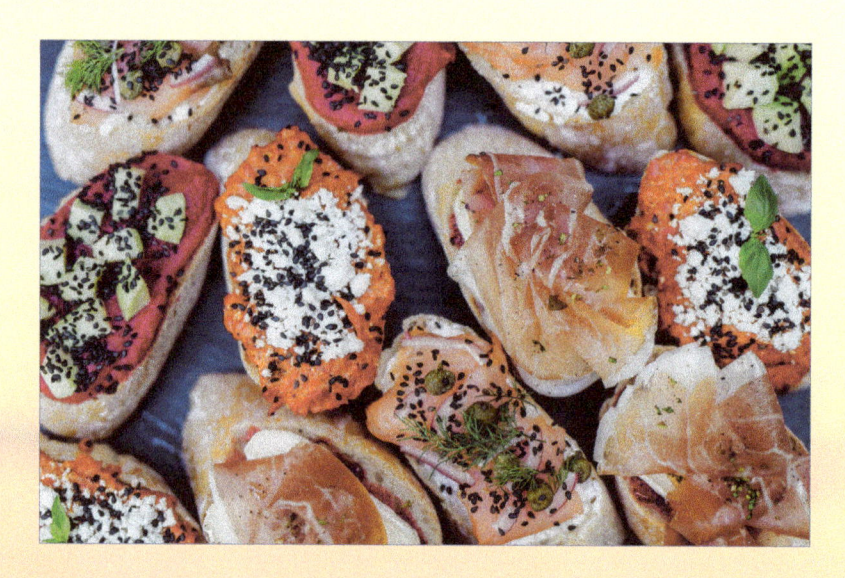

---

3. ESV

Chapter Ten

More Blessing...

Within a week following the event, have your teen write thank-you cards to all the guests and participants. This will not only further your efforts to instill a spirit of gratitude, but will give him or her an opportunity to review the events, cards, spoken words and gifts.

Over the course of the following months, during times of discouragement or confusion, review the Scriptures from the event. Continue to reaffirm the encouragement shared regarding God's declared plans and purposes.

It will be helpful, if you videotaped the event, to pull it out from time to time and share memories from this pivotal, Rite of Passage life-event.

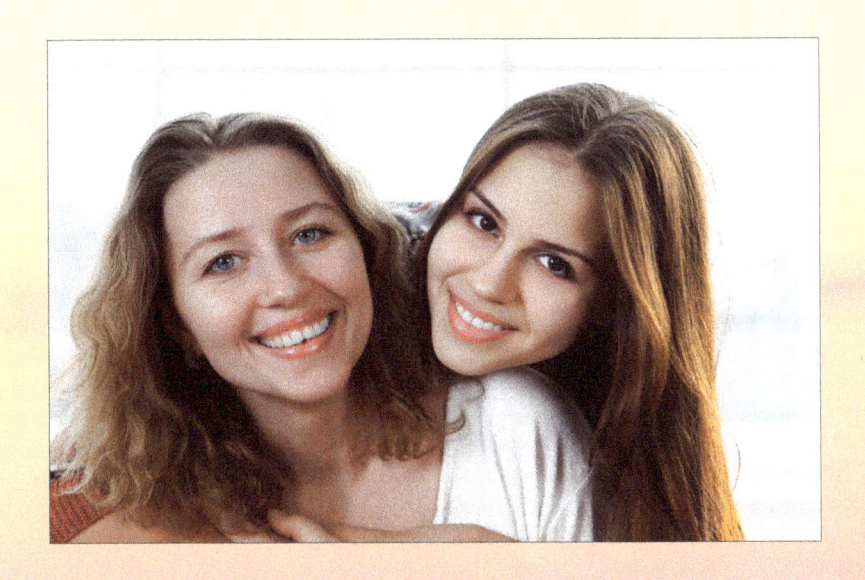

p. 44

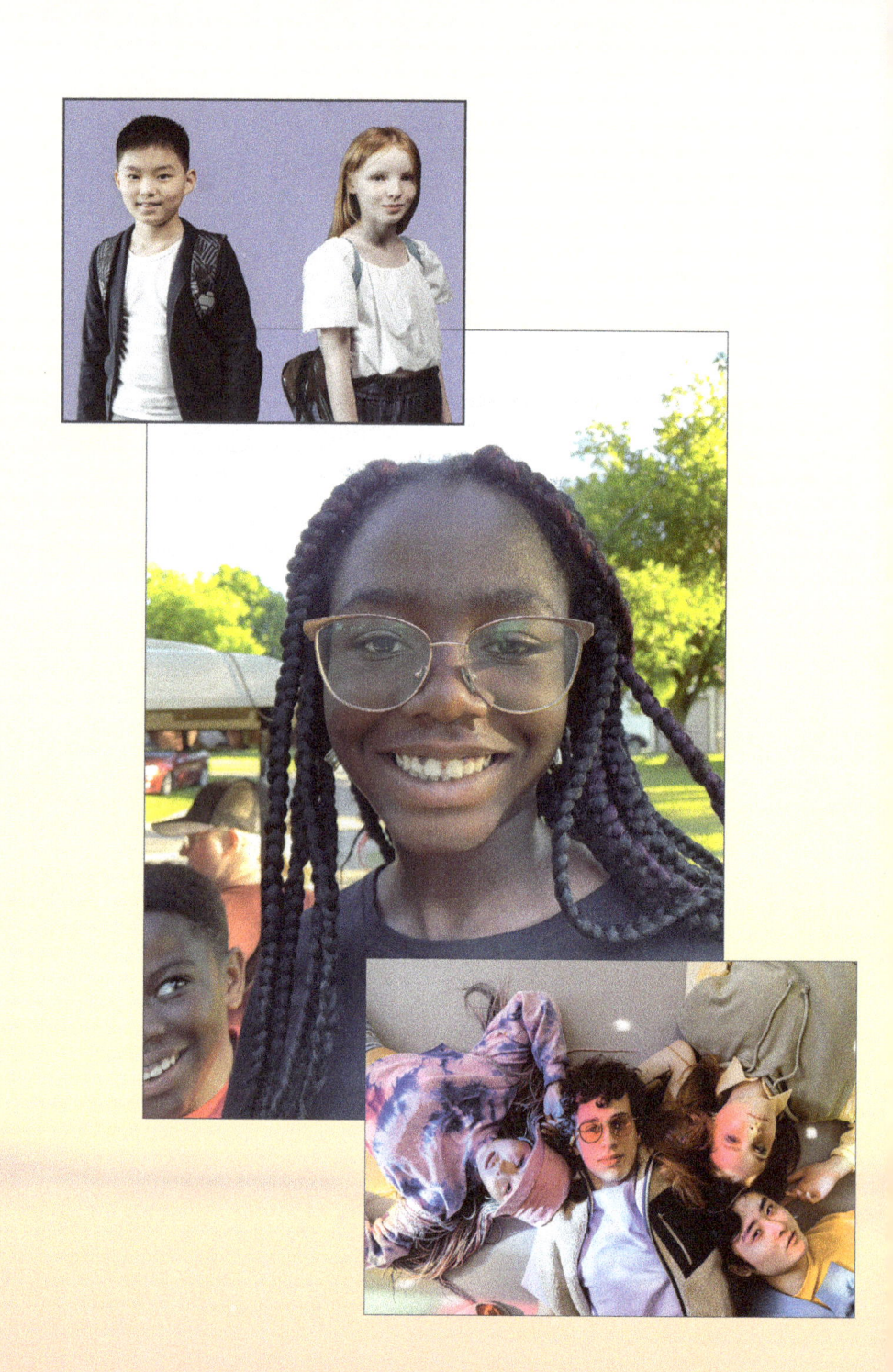

For Further Reading

Roblin-Lee, Diane, *The Family Blessing Initiative,* ByDesign Media, www.bydesignmedia.ca 110 East River Road, Paris, ON, 2010)

Hill, C. (2019) *The Power of a Parent's Blessing*, Charisma House.

Hill, C. (1998) *Bar Barakah: A Parent's Guide to a Christian Bar Mitzvah,* (Littleton, CO, Family Foundations Publishing, 1998)

Hill, C. *The Ancient Paths* (Littleton, CO, Family Foundations Publishing, 1992)

Hill, C. Raising Godly Children (3-Cassette Series, Littleton, CO, Family Foundations Publishing)

King, P. (2020) *The Power of a Decree*, Patricia King Enterprises.

Smalley, Gary and Trent, John, (2011) *The Blessing*, Nashville, Thomas Nelson, Inc. 1986.

Vanuaranu, Ari (2019) From Luxurious to Perilous, Here are some of the Most Fascinating Rites of Passage, *https:/The AseanPost.com*, Accessed Sept. 4, 2023.

"Thirteen Amazing Coming of Age Traditions From Around the World" www.globalcitizen.org, Accessed Sept. 4, 2023.

Swope, Mary Ruth (2009) *The Power of Blessing Your Children*, Christian Book Distributors.

Brodsky, Jeff, *Stepping Into Adulthood* (Phoenix, ACW Press, 1997)

Lewis, Robert, *Raising a Modern Day Knight* (Colorado Springs, Focus on the Family Publishing, 1997).

Ligon, WMT, *Imparting the Blessing to Your Children* (Workbook & 4-Cassette Series, Brunswick, Shalom, Inc., Box 1218, Brunswick GA 31521, 1989)

Durfield, R., & Durfield, Renee, *Raising them Chaste* (Minneapolis, Bethany House Publishers, 1991)

Anderson, Allie, *Unscrambling the Millennial Paradox* (Crane, MO 65633, Defender Publishing, 2019)

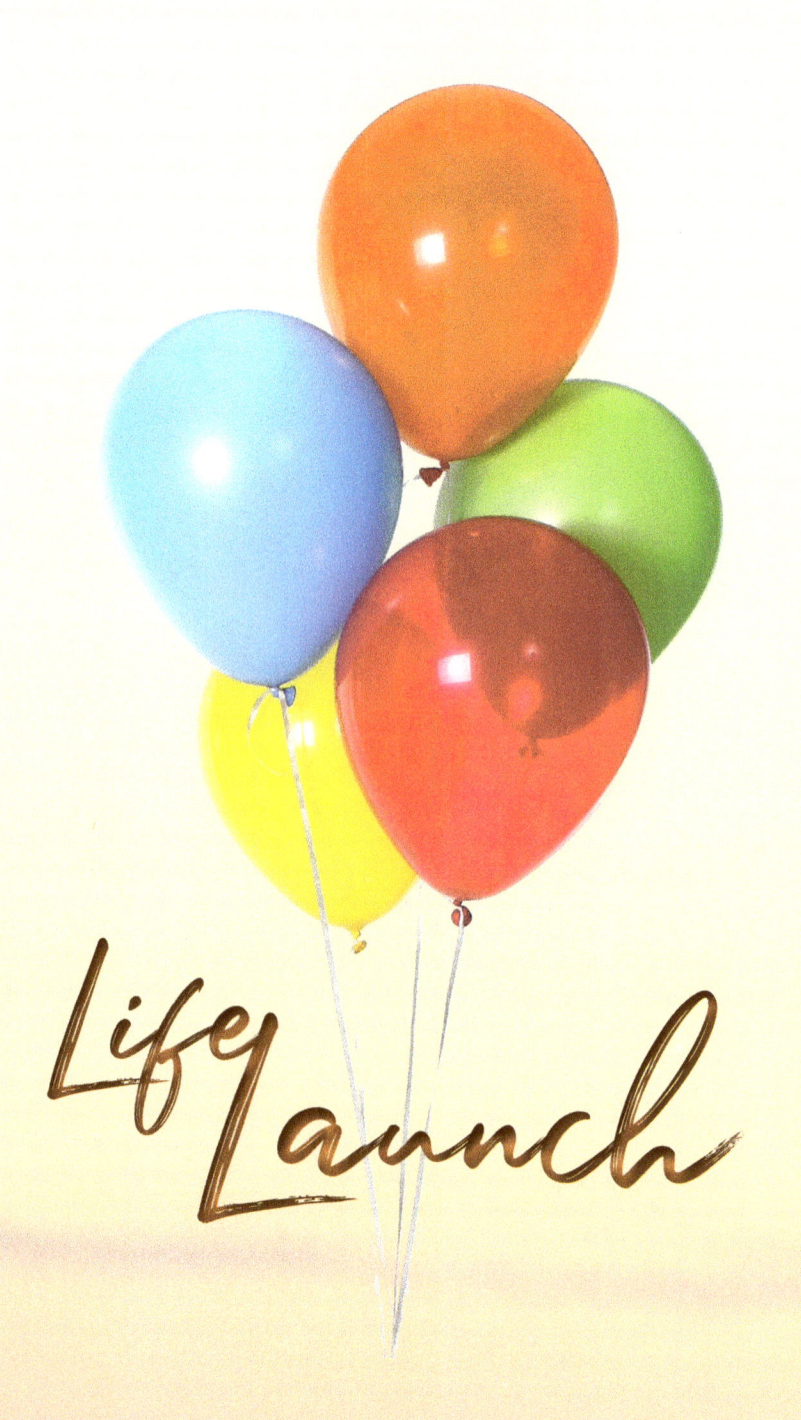

Life Launch

*You are Invited
to Join Us
in Celebrating the
LifeLaunch of*

_____

. . . as he /she crosses the threshold from childhood
into the next stage of his or her life journey.

As a valued member of our community
of family and special friends, your presence
will be very special to us.

If you have special words of memory or blessing you'd like to share,
please include them in a card or letter which will be treasured.

Date: _____
Time: _____
Location: _____
_____
RSVP by (Date): _____

p. 48

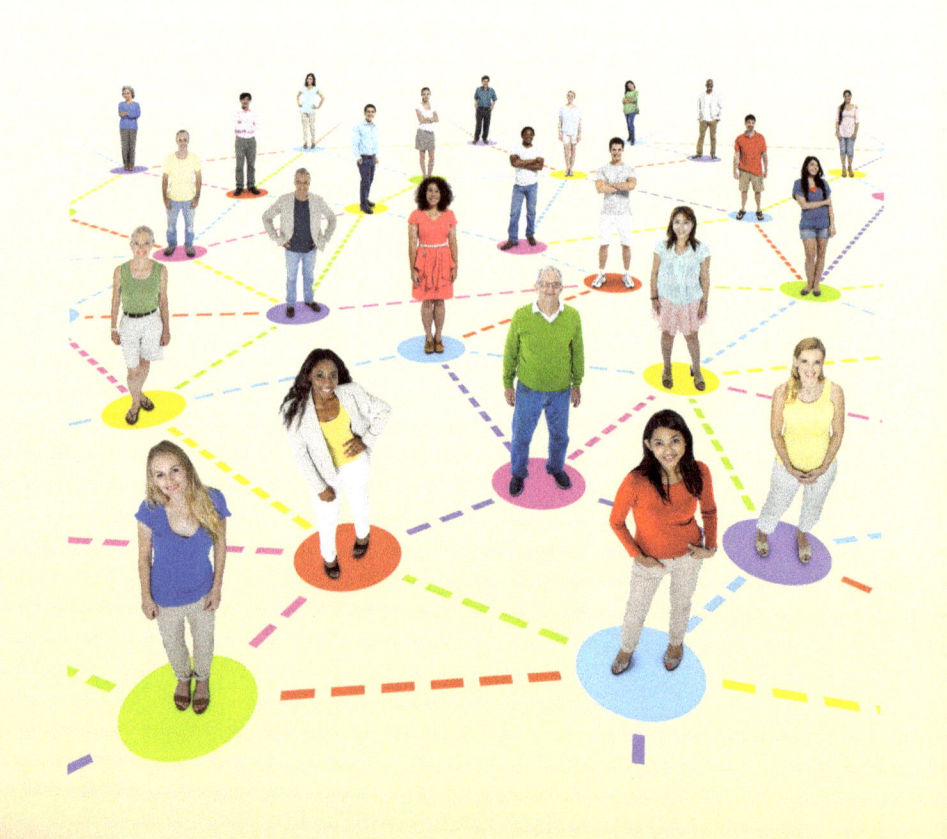

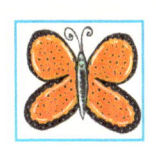

Invitations

Guest   Coming

Name
Address
Phone
E-mail
Note

Name
Address
Phone
E-mail
Note

Name
Address
Phone
E-mail
Note

Name
Address
Phone
E-mail
Note

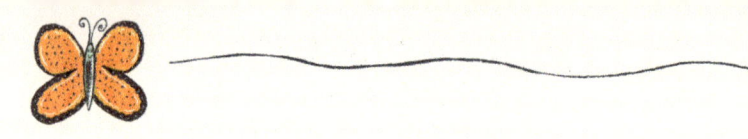

Invitations

Guest　　　　　　　　　　　　　　　　　　　Coming

Name
Address
Phone
E-mail
Note

Name
Address
Phone
E-mail
Note

Name
Address
Phone
E-mail
Note

Name
Address
Phone
E-mail
Note

Invitations

Guest	Coming
Name	
Address	
Phone	
E-mail	
Note	

Name
Address
Phone
E-mail
Note

Name
Address
Phone
E-mail
Note

Name
Address
Phone
E-mail
Note

Invitations

Guest — Coming

- Name
- Address
- Phone
- E-mail
- Note

- Name
- Address
- Phone
- E-mail
- Note

- Name
- Address
- Phone
- E-mail
- Note

- Name
- Address
- Phone
- E-mail
- Note

Invitations

Guest	Coming
Name	
Address	
Phone	
E-mail	
Note	

Name
Address
Phone
E-mail
Note

Name
Address
Phone
E-mail
Note

Name
Address
Phone
E-mail
Note

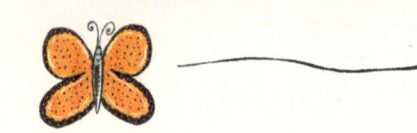

Invitations

Guest	Coming
Name	
Address	
Phone	
E-mail	
Note	
Name	
Address	
Phone	
E-mail	
Note	
Name	
Address	
Phone	
E-mail	
Note	
Name	
Address	
Phone	
E-mail	
Note	

Invitations

Guest   Coming

- Name
- Address
- Phone
- E-mail
- Note

- Name
- Address
- Phone
- E-mail
- Note

- Name
- Address
- Phone
- E-mail
- Note

- Name
- Address
- Phone
- E-mail
- Note

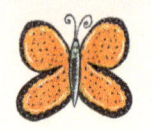

Invitations

Guest   Coming

Name
Address
Phone
E-mail
Note

Name
Address
Phone
E-mail
Note

Name
Address
Phone
E-mail
Note

Name
Address
Phone
E-mail
Note

Invitations

| Guest | Coming |

Name
Address
Phone
E-mail
Note

Name
Address
Phone
E-mail
Note

Name
Address
Phone
E-mail
Note

Name
Address
Phone
E-mail
Note

Invitations

Guest	Coming

Name
Address
Phone
E-mail
Note

Name
Address
Phone
E-mail
Note

Name
Address
Phone
E-mail
Note

Name
Address
Phone
E-mail
Note

Invitations

Guest   Coming

Name
Address
Phone
E-mail
Note

Name
Address
Phone
E-mail
Note

Name
Address
Phone
E-mail
Note

Name
Address
Phone
E-mail
Note

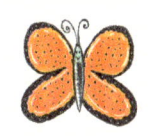

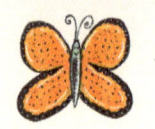

Invitations

Guest	Coming
Name	
Address	
Phone	
E-mail	
Note	

Name
Address
Phone
E-mail
Note

Name
Address
Phone
E-mail
Note

Name
Address
Phone
E-mail
Note

Invitations

Guest	Coming

Name
Address
Phone
E-mail
Note

Name
Address
Phone
E-mail
Note

Name
Address
Phone
E-mail
Note

Name
Address
Phone
E-mail
Note

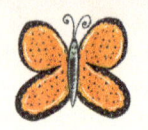

Invitations

Guest	Coming
Name	
Address	
Phone	
E-mail	
Note	
Name	
Address	
Phone	
E-mail	
Note	
Name	
Address	
Phone	
E-mail	
Note	
Name	
Address	
Phone	
E-mail	
Note	

Invitations

Guest   Coming

Name
Address
Phone
E-mail
Note

Name
Address
Phone
E-mail
Note

Name
Address
Phone
E-mail
Note

Name
Address
Phone
E-mail
Note

Invitations

Guest	Coming
Name	
Address	
Phone	
E-mail	
Note	

Name
Address
Phone
E-mail
Note

Name
Address
Phone
E-mail
Note

Name
Address
Phone
E-mail
Note

Invitations

Guest   Coming

Name
Address
Phone
E-mail
Note

Name
Address
Phone
E-mail
Note

Name
Address
Phone
E-mail
Note

Name
Address
Phone
E-mail
Note

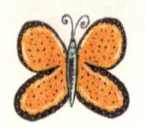

Invitations

Guest · Coming

Name
Address
Phone
E-mail
Note

Name
Address
Phone
E-mail
Note

Name
Address
Phone
E-mail
Note

Name
Address
Phone
E-mail
Note

Invitations

Guest   Coming

Name
Address
Phone
E-mail
Note

Name
Address
Phone
E-mail
Note

Name
Address
Phone
E-mail
Note

Name
Address
Phone
E-mail
Note

Invitations

Guest   Coming

Name
Address
Phone
E-mail
Note

Name
Address
Phone
E-mail
Note

Name
Address
Phone
E-mail
Note

Name
Address
Phone
E-mail
Note

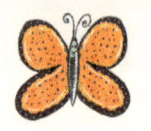

Invitations

Guest	Coming

Name
Address
Phone
E-mail
Note

Name
Address
Phone
E-mail
Note

Name
Address
Phone
E-mail
Note

Name
Address
Phone
E-mail
Note

Invitations

Guest   Coming

Name
Address
Phone
E-mail
Note

Name
Address
Phone
E-mail
Note

Name
Address
Phone
E-mail
Note

Name
Address
Phone
E-mail
Note

Invitations

Guest	Coming

Name
Address
Phone
E-mail
Note

Name
Address
Phone
E-mail
Note

Name
Address
Phone
E-mail
Note

Name
Address
Phone
E-mail
Note

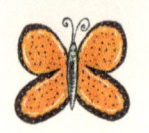

Invitations

Guest — **Coming**

Name
Address
Phone
E-mail
Note

Name
Address
Phone
E-mail
Note

Name
Address
Phone
E-mail
Note

Name
Address
Phone
E-mail
Note

Invitations

Guest   Coming

Name
Address
Phone
E-mail
Note

Name
Address
Phone
E-mail
Note

Name
Address
Phone
E-mail
Note

Name
Address
Phone
E-mail
Note

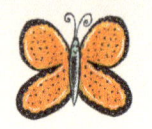

Invitations

Guest   Coming

- Name
- Address
- Phone
- E-mail
- Note

- Name
- Address
- Phone
- E-mail
- Note

- Name
- Address
- Phone
- E-mail
- Note

- Name
- Address
- Phone
- E-mail
- Note

Invitations

Guest | Coming

Name
Address
Phone
E-mail
Note

Name
Address
Phone
E-mail
Note

Name
Address
Phone
E-mail
Note

Name
Address
Phone
E-mail
Note

Invitations

Guest	Coming

Name
Address
Phone
E-mail
Note

Name
Address
Phone
E-mail
Note

Name
Address
Phone
E-mail
Note

Name
Address
Phone
E-mail
Note

Invitations

Guest	Coming

Name
Address
Phone
E-mail
Note

Name
Address
Phone
E-mail
Note

Name
Address
Phone
E-mail
Note

Name
Address
Phone
E-mail
Note

Invitations

Guest	Coming
Name	
Address	
Phone	
E-mail	
Note	
Name	
Address	
Phone	
E-mail	
Note	
Name	
Address	
Phone	
E-mail	
Note	
Name	
Address	
Phone	
E-mail	
Note	

Invitations

Guest	Coming
Name	
Address	
Phone	
E-mail	
Note	

Name
Address
Phone
E-mail
Note

Name
Address
Phone
E-mail
Note

Name
Address
Phone
E-mail
Note

p. 80

Guest Book

Guest Book

Name
Note

Name
Note

Name
Note

Name
Note

Guest Book

Name
Note

Name
Note

Name
Note

Name
Note

Guest Book

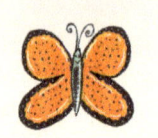

Name

Note

Name

Note

Name

Note

Name

Note

Guest Book

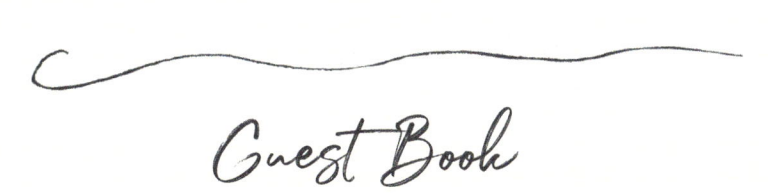

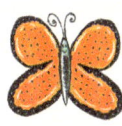

Name
Note

Name
Note

Name
Note

Name
Note

Guest Book

Name
Note

Name
Note

Name
Note

Name
Note

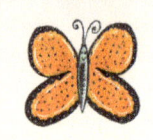

Guest Book

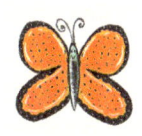

Name

Note

Name

Note

Name

Note

Name

Note

Guest Book

Name
Note

Name
Note

Name
Note

Name
Note

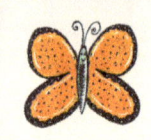

Guest Book

Name
Note

Name
Note

Name
Note

Name
Note

Guest Book

Name
Note

Name
Note

Name
Note

Name
Note

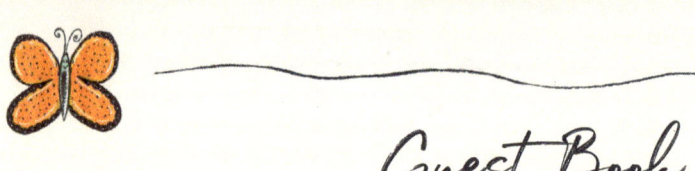

Guest Book

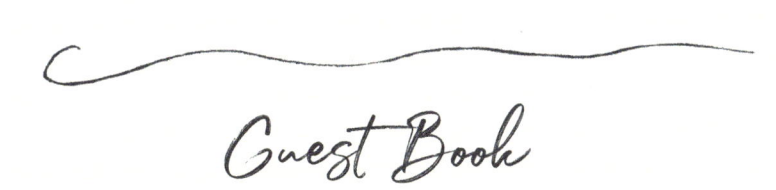

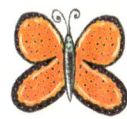

Name
Note

Name
Note

Name
Note

Name
Note

Guest Book

Name
Note

Name
Note

Name
Note

Name
Note

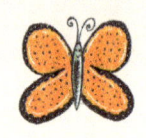

Guest Book

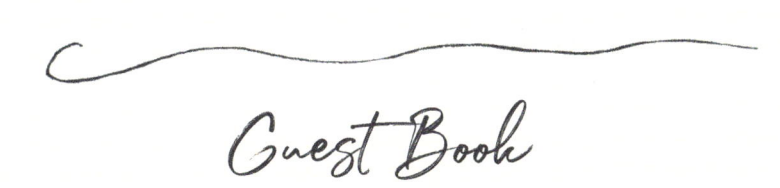

Name
Note

Name
Note

Name
Note

Name
Note

Guest Book

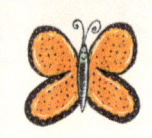

Name
Note

Name
Note

Name
Note

Name
Note

Guest Book

Name
Note

Name
Note

Name
Note

Name
Note

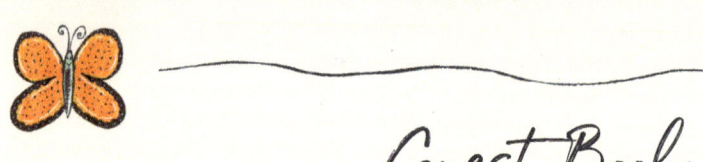

Guest Book

Name _____
Note _____
_____
_____

Name _____
Note _____
_____
_____

Name _____
Note _____
_____
_____

Name _____
Note _____
_____
_____

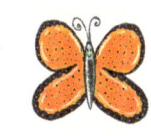

Guest Book

Name
Note

Name
Note

Name
Note

Name
Note

Guest Book

Name
Note

Name
Note

Name
Note

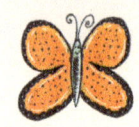

Name
Note

Guest Book

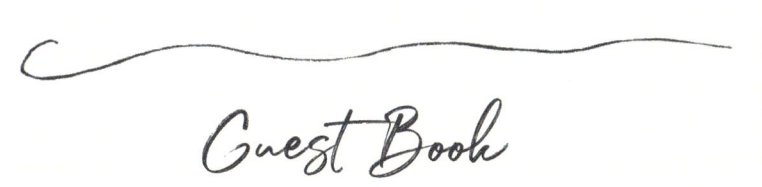

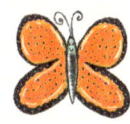

Name _____
Note _____
_____
_____
_____

Name _____
Note _____
_____
_____
_____

Name _____
Note _____
_____
_____
_____

Name _____
Note _____
_____
_____
_____

Guest Book

Name

Note

Name

Note

Name

Note

Name

Note

Guest Book

Name
Note

Name
Note

Name
Note

Name
Note

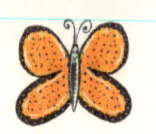

Guest Book

Name
Note

Name
Note

Name
Note

Name
Note

Guest Book

Name
Note

Name
Note

Name
Note

Name
Note

Guest Book

Name
Note

Name
Note

Name
Note

Name
Note

Guest Book

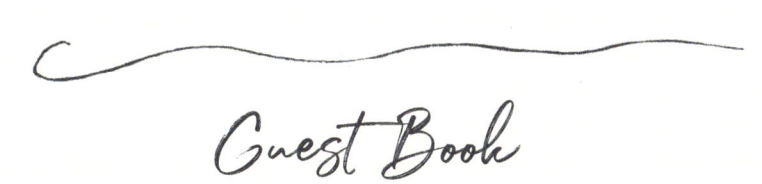

Name
Note

Name
Note

Name
Note

Name
Note

Guest Book

Name

Note

Name

Note

Name

Note

Name

Note

Guest Book

Name

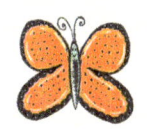

Note

Name

Note

Name

Note

Name

Note

Guest Book

Name
Note

Name
Note

Name
Note

Name
Note

Guest Book

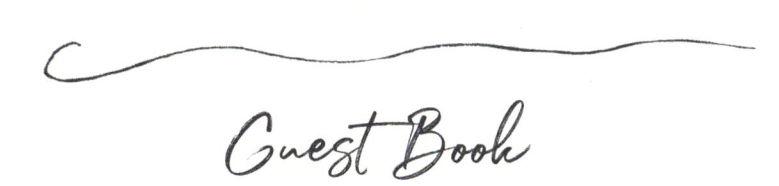

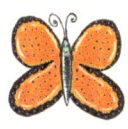

Name
Note

Name
Note

Name
Note

Name
Note

LifeNet4Hope.com

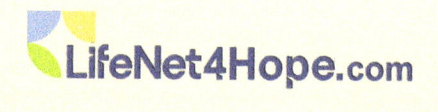

www.lifenet-lifelaunch.com

Printed in the USA
CPSIA information can be obtained
at www.ICGtesting.com
JSHW010010240923
48893JS00007BA/27